Insulin Resistance Strategies

Strategies to Overcome Insulin Resistance, Control Blood Sugar and Lose Weight

The information herein is offered for informational purposes solely, and is universal as so. The presentation of the information is without contract or any type of guarantee assurance.

Matthew Ward

Table of Contents

Introduction

As a growing national concern, insulin resistance ultimately progresses to diabetes if gone unchecked. Most resources implicate that it affects 18 to 21 million Americans, and still five to six million people are not aware of it yet. That's why learning about it is the first step toward reversal. It has been revealed that diabetes is the sixth leading cause of death in the United States, with one and a half million people diagnosed each year.

Researchers account obesity and an inactive lifestyle to these figures. While these factors definitely contribute to diabetes, you will come to be aware of the stealthy underlying influences from this book that pioneering doctors and researchers are discovering as they learn more about just how the body works.

This book contains proven steps and strategies on how to identify the signs and symptoms of insulin resistance, help source the cause of the issue, and monitor your blood sugar to keep your levels within a normal range. With a dedicated effort, these proven strategies can help you or a loved one move forward from the wakeup call that has brought you to this crossroads.

Well-rounded and complete, this book will provide you with the basics of blood sugar maintenance, encompassing full-scale diet and exercise layouts, just to give you an idea. You will also find palliative info about still basic yet less obvious influences on reversing insulin resistance. Such examples include the importance of quality sleep, the depth and magnitude of stress factors, water intake and effective natural supplements; all ultimately mapping out a comprehensive understanding of how we are put together as dynamic living beings.

It boils down to a clear and thorough regimen of navigating this life in a way that helps you feel your best by your own means. Deep down we all know what personally works for us and what doesn't when we listen to our bodies and that inner conscience that wants the best for us. Oftentimes external guidance, like road signs on the path of life, helps to direct and redirect us toward those well-intentioned goals in the midst of unfamiliar territory.

Your exploration of this book has brought your search here for a reason. Whether recognizing the need for a change in yours or someone else's life, simply looking for more proactive information about insulin resistance or otherwise, it is a sign. You can sense it in one way or another and this book has been designed with that sympathetic mentality. Rest assured that you will be provided with the key facts and identifiers you need to know, supplemental information you will want know, and relevant tips that perhaps you are not aware of yet.

Chapter 1: What is Insulin Resistance?

Let's start with the root of what we are talking about here. Insulin, a natural regulating hormone in the body, is produced by specialized cells in the pancreas known as 'beta cells'. It promotes tissue cells in the body (muscles, skin, organs, etc.) to uptake glucose, a broken-down form of what we know as sugar, so that they may use it for energy to keep functioning properly. A side job of insulin is to help remove fat from blood and usher it into fat storage cells.

Now comparatively, while nerve cells and their impulses transmit feedback information within the body to the brain instantly, hormone feedback takes much longer because it is carried through bloodwork. That means that hormone regulation is a slow process that produces traceable results within a matter of hours while significant medical testing looks at reliable figures over weeks and months.

The common index that doctors use to determine if a person is insulin resistant is called 'A1c'. A person's A1C looks at average hemoglobin or blood sugar levels from the past three months prior to bloodwork tests. A healthy person's A1C index number should register between 4% and 5.9%, while anything at 8% or more glucose in the blood suggests insulin resistance.

Insulin Resistance

So what does being 'insulin resistant 'imply? Synonymous with the term diabetes, it reveals that glucose and fats build up in the bloodstream either because the beta cells of the pancreas decrease or cease insulin production altogether, insulin receptors in the tissue cells of the body develop a resistance to accepting the hormone, or both.

When this happens a host of issues occur. Blood sugar levels rise, stimulating further insulin production (the body's normal reaction); in the case of insulin resistance, some beta cells are still functioning and tissue cell receptors are inhibited. This leads to hyperglycemia (too much sugar in the blood) and hyperinsulinemia (excessive insulin levels in the blood) at the same time, which introduces the body to the onset of type 2 diabetes.

Further disorders result from the above situation such as an increased risk of heart disease, overloaded abdominal fat cells, and dysfunction or failure of other organs like the kidneys, bladder and liver. Abdominal fat cells function differently than what we think of in terms of fat: metabolically (converting glucose and other sources into energy), they produce several chemicals that have hostile effects on body functions. Along with that, the accumulation of blood sugars breaks down cell function, bathing the surrounding tissues.

Consider the kidneys, our vital organs that filter the blood, which become overtaxed; the bladder, which disposes the excess waste of the body and in an untreated diabetic person can show traceable amounts of sugar content; the liver, another vital organ that plays jack of all trades in terms of functional purposes, including the breakdown of red blood cells at the end of their lifetime. A crucial role of the liver recycles some of the red blood cells' components, such as the structure that provides the ability to carry oxygen to every cell of the body. We will cover further adverse effects of untreated insulin resistance later on. First, we will explore the two main varieties of diabetes that are commonly seen.

Like heart disease, insulin resistance is often a silent disorder, so it is difficult to know if one has it unless they are tested. This can be done a few ways: one way to identify it is by testing blood glucose and/or insulin after fasting when these levels should be low. A more direct test used by other specialists measures blood glucose two hours after a person consumes 75 mg or roughly one-fifth of a teaspoon of sugar. Again, a healthy person should be unaffected by this dose and present a hemoglobin range of anywhere from 80 to 110, while an insulin resistant person will test a higher number. This test is more significant for catching the disorder early on.

Type 1 Diabetes

The onset of diabetes is usually seen as either type 1 or type 2, accounting for 98% of diagnoses. Type 1 diabetes is an autoimmune disorder, developing from any number of triggers including certain drugs and chemicals, some types of infections, and a family history of the condition. It is labeled as 'autoimmune' because immune cells of the body specifically attack beta cells. Currently in mainstream medicine there is no cure for this type, leading to lifelong insulin deficiency and dependence externally. That makes it considerably more serious than type 2 diabetes however it is rare as well.

Type 1 usually reveals symptoms before the age of 30, so it is easier to catch and start receiving treatment early on in life. Because the beta cells have been killed off by the immune system, it becomes a daily responsibility to closely monitor one's activities which reduce blood sugars, their diet which can raise blood sugars at every bite, and the self-administered insulin doses to keep these levels in check. The body will have no ability to self-regulate, so with type 1 blood levels can fluctuate in extremes when not in careful check: polarities include levels high enough to cause ketoacidosis and diabetic coma to low enough that they lead to epileptic seizures from insulin shock.

Type 2 Diabetes

This is the most common form of diabetes, largely developing within people who become obese or lead relatively inactive lifestyles. In fact, roughly 90% of people with this type are overweight when diagnosed. The good news about this type is that in most cases, many who get it will see symptoms disappear and the disorder reverse itself by losing weight to reach normal BMI levels.

Exactly how this type of insulin resistance comes about currently remains a mystery because it depends on the individual. Some develop it because of a high-carbohydrate diet that eventually wears down pancreatic function. Others may have normal insulin production but the glucose influx proves to be too much to handle or the cells in their body that should be receiving insulin have too few receptor sites. On the other hand, alternative risk factors include metabolic syndrome, immune system issues and increased blood clotting.

The bottom line is that there are so many factors that can weigh in results of diabetic symptoms and the disorder is still being understood while doctors' current vantage point is numbers-based, leading them to diagnose based on symptoms and blood sugars alone. There are still other factors to be considered that can lead to insulin resistance reversal as forefront medical experts are finding out when incorporating psychological and emotional aspects with bodily dysfunction.

This holistic approach sees each part intimately connected with the other and aims to get to the root of the dysfunction, going beyond simply addressing physical symptoms. As doctors are learning, oftentimes physical symptoms are the last manifestation of a medical disorder and the accumulation of stress in one's life usually ushers in a deeper understanding of the core issue where the disorder can be nipped in the bud. In this light, reversal of type 2 diabetes sees greater success with certain lifestyle changes particular to the individual.

Untreated Insulin Resistance

Emergencies to consider with insulin resistance are serious and can be deadly if not properly cared for immediately. Reviewing these will reveal a few important themes pertaining to the nature of our bodies and the environment that affects them, namely pH levels. Another theme that has briefly been mentioned before and will continue to be discussed throughout this book because of its central relevance is the issue of stress and/or emotional trauma.

Our bodies optimally function at a pH level just above neutral of 7.1, being slightly basic or alkaline, while anything below 7 is acidic on the pH scale. This is a generic, all-encompassing number since we can find different pH levels occurring within different parts of the body.

It may interest you to know that certain foods like carbohydrates and especially sugar turns the body's pH levels acidic while other foods such as vegetables, especially root vegetables, and dark leafy greens, will help to alkalize the body. Maintaining a more alkaline-based diet and environment within the body is important. It has been found that an acidic body opens the gates for bacteria, pathogens, illnesses and even cancers to potentially thrive while they cannot survive in an alkaline environment. More about this will be covered in chapter 4 on food groups.

Ketoacidosis is the medical emergency case in which there is a crucial lack of insulin and glucose in the cells of type 1 diabetics and only people with type 1. The body partially converts fats into energy, emitting an acidic byproduct of that metabolism called ketones that drastically changes the pH balance of the blood. A sweet or fruity odor on the breath is one way to detect this condition. Another way is to purchase test strips that measure ketone levels in the urine. This critical condition arises from various factors such as stress, infection or trauma and can amplify to shock, coma, and death.

In type 2 diabetes, the increased concentration of sugars in the blood as a solution ratio to the water in our bodies can reach exceeding levels that result in something known as *hyperosmolality*. Due to such high blood sugar levels, the body's pH levels turn gravely acidic and like ketoacidosis can result in shock, coma, and death.

On the other end of the spectrum, considering that insulin resistance involves an insulin imbalance that entails both too high or too low blood sugars, the latter situation can lead up to *insulin shock*. This means there is too much insulin in the bloodstream caused by a few reasons. A diabetic person could have administered too much insulin, or such factors like a skipped meal, sudden exertion, stress, infection, or trauma cause the body to metabolize all blood sugar resources. Too much insulin means very low blood sugars, known as hypoglycemia. The symptoms to watch out for in this case are dizziness, confusion, weakness in the muscles, and tremors. This case also leads to potential coma and death if gone untreated.

Chapter 2: Be Aware of the Signs and Symptoms

Between type 1 and type 2 diabetes among the other types, you may find yourself confused as how to accurately detect the signs when insulin resistance can ultimately occur at any stage in life. Rest assured that while several factors may induce its onset and many symptoms can result from it, diabetes produces specific 'tells' that you can watch out for and consult a professional about if they appear for you or a family member.

There are three basic signs that are characteristic to the onset of all types of diabetes known as the "polys". *Polyuria* refers to frequent urination above normal that is caused by elevated blood sugar; as opposed to salt, which helps to retain water within the body, excess sugar draws water out of the body's cells and is then released in the urine. You will find that this also results in chronic dehydration, which leads right into the next 'poly'.

An important side note is that if you ever find yourself with dry mouth, diabetes or not, this is the last sign of dehydration that manifests in the body meaning that you have already been dehydrated for quite some time before this symptom showed up. It should be an indicator that you need to hydrate – that is, consume water and straight up *just water* – immediately.

Polydipsia is the condition of excessive thirst that is systemically linked to the loss of water with polyuria. If you find yourself or another reaching for a beverage more often than usual, or if indeed someone makes that observation about you, it should be an indicator to consider getting checked out.

Polyphagia denotes an increase in appetite. This results because the body's cells have trouble taking on glucose derived from the breakdown of digested carbohydrates. Unfortunately, these are the most effectual form of energy for the body, and in the case of diabetes the body must then convert fat stores for fuel, and after that is gone it resorts to protein (namely muscle tissues, causing them to atrophy in due time).

Symptoms deriving from these three "polys" lead to effects experienced as chronic fatigue of the body as well as mental processes, weight loss due to polyphagia and nausea and vomiting from polydipsia.

Remember that diabetes starts out subtly and silently, and while these signs might not seem like anything serious in the moment, they are often overlooked for that reason while the illness progresses to damage other organs. Just like any other serious disorder, the earlier on that it can be caught and get treated with the proper care the better. It will mean less time and work for the body to recover and stabilize, allowing you to get back into your life the way you love to live it with hopefully a healthier approach that continues to empower the quality of your daily experiences.

Complications of Diabetic Progression

Beyond the "polys" are more serious complications stemming from the progression of insulin resistance. They are more notable and obvious physical symptoms that often give way to one pursuing medical attention since the person has finally become aware of his or her state of disease, as in "out of a healthy comfort zone", by this time a little worse off for not catching it sooner. Listed below is an easy-to-read layout of these complications with explanations for each one.

Cardiovascular disease: Because high blood glucose levels cause an acidic change in pH, the insides of the veins and arteries and those of the heart get eaten away, damaged due to insulin resistance. Along with the associative increase of fat cells in the bloodstream, it becomes an open invitation for atherosclerosis. The complication here is that unlike the typical development of atherosclerosis within the artery walls alone, a diabetic patient will accumulate fatty plaque throughout the body. Stroke, hypertension (high blood pressure), and aneurysm (blood clotting and blockage of vessels) all become increased risks. This is the majority cause of death in people with diabetes at about two-thirds to three-quarters of the patient population.

Edema: meaning the swelling of some part of the body, happens because of a slow and lethargic blood in the veins. It can be found within the extremities, but the lower legs, ankles and feet of a diabetic person are usually where the swelling happens. Did you know that 70 percent of blood in the body is found in the legs at any given time? It is due to gravity as well as the fact that blood flow takes much longer in veins that return it to the heart than in arteries, which contain smooth muscle to help the blood flow out. Therefore, it greatly helps insulin resistant people with edema to keep their legs raised and resting as often as possible so that gravity works for them rather than against them.

Ulcers, gangrene and amputations: These highly undesirable effects result from an epidemic of plaque buildup throughout the entire circulatory network. Because blood flow is so drastically constrained many areas of the body, especially the furthest extremities such as the feet, our natural capacity to heal and regenerate cells becomes altogether ineffective. Even small cuts and scrapes can't heal; ingrown toenails, blisters, or pressure spots on the feet can turn into a life-threatening situation. Without blood reaching these areas, the cells can die from nutrient starvation or be at the mercy of infection and pathogens without white blood cells to fight off. This becomes a noticeable sign in the form of diabetic ulcers that are usually found on the soles of the feet where pressure is applied when standing and walking. Without care, diabetes has become the reason for about 82,000 lower extremity amputations each year.

Kidney disease: The kidneys are the filtration system for all the blood that consistently runs throughout our entire body. They are also one of the first branches of the descending aorta and thus become clogged with plaque very easily. Polyuria, the constant urination symptom of diabetes that starts with the kidneys, taxes their function by causing them to work harder and can lead up to renal failure and the need for transplants.

Impaired vision: Our eyes contain millions of very tiny capillaries, which you can see usually if you have ever missed a night's sleep or swam in a pool with too much chlorine. Diabetes will thicken these blood vessels, leaving the eyes without necessary nutrition, creating a risk of microaneurysms, and leaking blood and proteins into the retina. The exorbitant amount of sugar in the blood can bind to proteins in the lens of the eye causing cataracts and eventually blindness. This issue is the leading cause of new blindness in people from 20 to 70 years old in the U.S.

Neuropathy: As it has been mentioned, tissues that are bathed in a highly sugary solution of blood become weakened, damaged, and eaten away at in this acidic environment. Along with absent capillary circulation, this leads to nerve damage experienced by sensations of tingling, pain, and numbness. When neuropathy hits the central nervous system (brain, brainstem, and spinal cord), the ability to maintain blood pressure becomes unstable, as well as a number of other automated systems in the body: delayed or inefficient emptying of the stomach, diarrhea, constipation and sexual impotency. This usually occurs somewhere between 10 and 20 years after diabetes is diagnosed, so people with the illness who maintain it well from diagnosis and alter their lifestyle to attempt reversal are unlikely to reach this point.

Others: Since diabetes directly involves the circulatory system and all cells in the body interact with the blood as a necessary means of functioning, pretty much every body system becomes affected by diabetes. This is why the symptoms are so wide-ranging. The disorder is also connected to UTIs, candidiasis, birth defects, aggressive ear infections that can invade the skull, and abnormal rates of gingivitis and tooth loss.

Chapter 3: Take a Stand, Make a Turn Around

Stand up, sit down, crunch and kick! Go for a run, swim in place, make the exercise stick!

So, enough of the scary stuff. Now that you know what to look out for and just how serious diabetes can be, hopefully, you will never have to encounter a case that gets that bad. Education, prevention, and responsible maintenance are steady steps toward positive relief from dealing with this illness. Spread the word and share the information with your loved ones.

Keeping an uplifted mentality and motivation to move past the stipulations of insulin resistance will also help the recovery process, so don't ever let anyone say that you or they are stuck with diabetes. Let's look at the options there are before us to start turning insulin resistance into a healthy flow of confidence. For example, will losing weight help solve this problem?

When we think of losing weight, our minds are drawn to concepts of exercise. The sensation of that New Year's effort of bringing ourselves to the gym brings a micro boost of motivation into the lungs and we prepare ourselves for the long, steady climb ahead, usually falling short after a month or so after not seeing significant results.

Well, dredge not for reserves of stimulation, there is a new motivation afoot and it might just come from a direction that hasn't been considered yet. This isn't about looking good, it is about *feeling* good within the body and the mind. It is about embracing the life we *want* to live rather than living up to an image we may think we should embody. This is our health we're talking about!

Would you or someone you know rather cope with the constant maintenance of the insulin resistant predicament that has been reached, doing the tango of two steps forward and one step back as blood sugars are monitored, or would you like to take the assured, proactive steps in keeping those levels steady and progressively stabilizing with an edging smile of confidence?

The very first sentences of this chapter are a bit misleading to illustrate a point and really drive home some of the principles of the body reflected through the diabetic position. Exercise and physical exertion have their place in the recovery regimen, however in the practice of monitoring blood glucose levels, it is crucial to know that any mild to strenuous activity is going to cause those levels to drop. One must be careful to know where their levels are at before engaging in such activities in order to avoid them dropping too low and risking insulin shock.

The fact is there are other significant ways to lose weight that are equally if not more effective than exercise. This is important to know in the case of people with type 2 diabetes, especially if the gain of excess weight has caused them to become obese and onset the disorder in the first place. Many overweight people have found that with a shift in their diet alone, they were dropping pounds faster than an overloaded barbell. Food helped cause the problem, and

15

likewise, it can help to be the solution. The emphasis is on *what kinds of food the body responds well to* and *portion size.*

Proper nutrition sees to it that we are providing the body with its needs rather than its wants and cravings and within volumes that it is capable of handling. Providing the right portions at mealtimes will train the body to regulate itself again; not have to work as hard at digestion, whose ability and quality to process food is a major determiner of our overall health; and get the most out of what we feed ourselves with no great expenditure on waste production. Symptoms like acid indigestion, gassiness and bloating will phase out, and any foul odors produced by the body (commonly traced to sugar and stress caused by various reasons) will become neutralized.

Without feigning, this process indeed will take time and a fair amount of discipline to see it through but it does not have to be a struggle. On the contrary, within the first week, you will begin noticing results from an overall improvement in mood to the reduction and relief of some physical symptoms, as well as feeling *good* in your body. Essentially you will be treating your body with what it *needs* and it will be thanking you for it.

Many people who have changed up their diet to appropriately suit their body's needs have seen weight loss results. Because we are more than just our bodies, encompassing the regular mode of our emotional state that is reflected by the inhibiting or embracing thoughts that we have and indeed, our personal perspective by which we see the world. These new discoveries by researchers are making it more apparent of just how deep and interwoven our mindset and emotional states are with governing the state of our body's health, which in turn reflects the health of the first two.

A psychological study was conducted in the early 2000's on hotel maids, many of whom were overweight, pertaining to weight loss and the awareness of the activities they did in their work. They were interviewed and monitored individually and their daily home, work, and eating habits were all documented. Then the focus group of maids was divided in two, group A and group B. Group B was left as a control group to continue with their tasks unaltered by the study. Group A, however, was presented information so rudimentary that it is mesmerizing how deeply it affected them to produce the results that were observed. It unveiled certain truths about how dynamically we are put together that can and will be studied for decades to come.

Group A was told not to change any of their eating or home habits for the next few months, which across the board were mildly active to relatively sedentary outside of their work. The group was then questioned and presented with the information by the researchers, asking the maids if they were aware that the work they were doing in the hotels was actually exercise. Most all of them answered 'no'. Basic tasks like emptying garbage pails, changing bed sheets, cleaning bathrooms and vacuuming rooms were just considered to be part of the job.

The researchers then presented the group with an outline of how many calories each task burned within the body as they were performed and asked the maids to keep this in mind while they were working for the next few months. Ultimately, after this course of time most all of the maids were observed to experience some amount of weight loss, from a few pounds up to 20 pounds. Group B, on the other hand, had not seen much of any changes in their weight.

The maids in group A had not gone to the gym or changed their lifestyle except for an increase in the awareness of their actions and the effect it has on the body. This example has been brought to you to illustrate an important concept that will greatly accelerate your healing process and overall quality of life, which also pertains to the laws of attraction. The mind tells the body what to do both consciously and unconsciously, and with practice and awareness, we can learn to control our thoughts to create a new state of living for ourselves.

Controlling and reversing insulin resistance starts with nutrition. Changing the diet to incorporate nourishing foods for the body will help to change its internal environment that will, in turn, promote gradual weight loss. It will also prime the body and the mind to relax into a healthier state that makes the ensuing recovery process all the easier. Who knows, you or a loved one might just find yourselves having FUN with it, knowing that you are healing, taking back control of your life, and doing more to feel great about yourselves.

As for exercise, let's reiterate that vigorous activity only puts more strain on the body. That is not what a recovering body needs to improve health when the organs are already taxed and the potential of plaque buildup in the veins and arteries is a likelihood. This form of exercise we're talking about, which tends to be a common concept, raises the heart rate and blood circulation and causes the other organs such as the kidneys, lungs and liver to work harder. Not to say that cardio, aerobics, and weight training have their place down the road to recovery, and suggestions will be detailed in chapter 5, however, there are milder forms of activity to stimulate the body and meet its needs in a weakened state.

These exercises are characteristically slow, calm and controlled, so each repetition calls upon you to bring mindfulness in while doing them. Synchronizing the breath with the movement is another important aspect.

Why is this so important you may ask? It is straight logic: within movement, we are engaging the muscles to expand and contract. When we move slowly, we can focus more closely on performing the specific action with regard to good body mechanics, in turn promoting body awareness. Better body awareness prevents strain in motion and promotes better posture which removes strain on the muscles, internal organs, joints, and nerves.

This subsequently removes any stress on the mind; feeling good in the body means feeling good in the mind and more relaxed. As we relax with these slow exercises, we open up the blood flow in a healthy way to increase circulation. By synchronizing the breath with the movement, we are actively and consciously nurturing the blood and therefore the rest of the body, including the mind, with fresh oxygen. Filling the body with oxygen encourages the cells to relax more deeply and function properly. The reason illness is referred to as a "disease" is because the basic problem has stemmed from some sort of stress that has brought us out of a relaxed state of being over time and consistency.

To sum up, slow, controlled exercises with synchronized breath promote the body and mind with relief. They reduce stress and physical strain and create a more prominent environment for the body to heal, as is its natural and phenomenal ability. These types of exercises connect the mind and body to form a healthy relationship with each other, listen to each other's true needs, and work as one to allow you to focus on and live out your true desires and goals. As with anything worth doing and getting better at, it may not feel like much at first but with paced practice and consistency the results will speak for themselves.

Weight gain is related to a number of reasons, however, they can be traced back to the types of foods we eat, the portions, how active we are day to day, as well as how much stress we take on and *hold on* to. Think about how so many of us reach for fatty, salty, and/or sugary foods when we need a bit of comfort or relief. Think about, and really take the time to shed some awareness on this, the thoughts and mood we're absorbed in while we eat. Do we eat fast just to get something in our bodies, or do we take the time to really enjoy the meal and each bite?

In this sense, the body holds on to weight for a combination of the food nutritional content (or lack thereof) and accrued stress within the body. As we take steps to eat well and mindfully and combine them with exercises that filter out that accrued stress, promoting overall relaxation back into a state of mental and physical ease, the body responds by dropping the weight that was brought on by repetitive tension. The "disease" begins transforming back into a state of ease.

Chapter 4: Food Groups for the Insulin Resistant

If education is the first step to laying down a strong foundation of health then with consideration to insulin resistance, knowing about the impact of various foods on the body will pave the way toward the second step of creating a solid and reliable meal plan. In this chapter we will discuss various staple foods that are common in most balanced diets and how the components of each food group break down in the body, changing its internal environment. The chapter will also outline and highlight a tailored palate of foods from their components that are harmonious with an insulin resistant body system.

In order to get a good sense of where to start with a diabetic-friendly diet, let's first look at what we already know about the disorder and how it affects the body to calibrate finding suitable foods. We shall focus in on complex versus simple carbohydrates, the ever-underappreciated and underestimated power of the vegetable world and the value of proteins and fats. Another point of interest to be explored is the GI or *Glycemic Index*, which ranks carbohydrate-based foods by their impact on hemoglobin or blood glucose levels and references these with standard foods.

Carbohydrates

There are several foods across the board that contain carbohydrates to be aware of. We may typically think of breads, grains, pastas and so on as the carb heavy-hitters, and still there are many food sources grown in agriculture that are naturally carb-containing. Beans, rice, oats, potatoes, and corn are a few examples. Carbs are the most efficient source of fuel for the body's cells in order to optimally function so that we can be active and responsive throughout the day. So then it makes sense that so many foods, both cultivated and naturally grown, provide this vital nutrient for us to consume.

In a healthy person's body, after eating carb-containing foods the carbohydrates are broken down in the digestive system via the stomach, liver, and gall bladder. The result becomes a reserve of glucose which is then absorbed by the small intestine and drawn into the bloodstream so that it can be transported throughout the body along with oxygen and several other digested nutrients to sustain every cell in the body.

Messages are sent to the brain that an increase in hemoglobin levels have been introduced to the body and the brain sends messages back to the pancreas to produce insulin. Insulin is then released into the bloodstream as well, and acts like a key, binding to receptor sites in the cell walls that act like bodyguards to make sure that only good things are going into the cell and wastes are going out. When the insulin binds to these receptor sites they open up a "door" so to speak that has a specific shape unique to match the shape of glucose so that it can be admitted into the cell. Glucose being carried in the bloodstream is then delivered to these open doors in the cell walls and the cells absorb it and break it down further to be used as energy for the cells' internal processes.

Carbohydrates are the best fuel source for the body because, in comparison to fats or proteins, they break down the fastest in the process described above. That means relatively instant energy resources. So if someone feels fatigued, mentally slow or otherwise drained, eating carb-based foods will resupply them with new reserves of eventual energy to draw upon.

This is why you see hikers typically bring some assortment of trail mix containing oats, granola, nuts and so on. The same goes for power bars marketed to athletes and highly active people. However more and more often, unless you are shopping at a health-conscious store and sometimes even still, these packaged products are seasoned-to-taste with chocolate, candy pieces, and dried fruits that are preserved in refined sugar.

Added sugar in foods like those above provides a spike in energy temporarily but they burn up too quickly to be supportive. Because it requires energy from the body to process foods into energy, a sugar boost and burn up often leaves us feeling worse off afterward, also known as a "sugar crash". This same occurrence is seen in the consumption of simple carbohydrates as well. They break down quickly within the body but burn up too fast, leaving the person feeling fatigued one to three hours after eating. On top of that, both sugary foods and simple carbs cause a drastic rise in blood sugars.

In contrast, the sugar derivative of glucose obtained from the body processing complex carbs provides a slower burning of those energy reserves, making them much more sustainable. Complex carbs break down relatively slower than their simple counterparts, yet they are still a desirable fuel source for their sustainability factor. Complex carbs also have little to no effect on raising blood sugars, so they are an ideal resource for the insulin resistant person.

Such an afflicted person should still be leery of the effects of these types of foods on their blood sugar, so it is important when creating a diet that hemoglobin levels are monitored, tested and documented after eating such foods. Below you will find some common examples of foods containing simple and complex carbohydrates so that you may know the difference and use your discretion when formulating meal plans.

Simple carbs: White and yellow potatoes; most fruits and juices, even if they are 100% natural; white rice; any baked goods or pastas containing white flour; corn

Complex carbs: Most types of beans; sweet potatoes; multigrain and 100% whole wheat baked goods and pastas; berries; brown rice; oats (rolled, and especially steel-cut oats); quinoa; lentils

Vegetables

The all-hailed cream of the crop when it comes to reaping the benefits from food consumption, vegetables seemingly have a stigmatized reputation as being "weak" foods for some reason. Perhaps it is because of their earthy or neutral taste that just does not sit right on most people's tongues or it could because one just cannot sink their teeth into a vegetable the way they can with meat. Whatever the case may be, vegetable produce takes the carrot cake when it comes to hardy eating.

It is true in terms of energy resources that greater quantities of vegetables must be consumed and more frequently in order to match the levels that complex carbs or proteins provide. Be that as it may, vegetables provide a whole library of the necessary vitamins, minerals, fiber and nutrients that our bodies require in their wide-ranging world. Dark leafy greens like spinach, kale, and collard greens are rich in iron that supports the blood to efficiently carry oxygen to other cells throughout the body. Broccoli florets contain superior amounts of potassium over the commonly conceived banana, and that is a great supplement to support the nervous system.

Vegetables also support the body in a significant way that few other foods are capable of doing. Because they grow in soils that are rich in minerals, they are primarily alkaline. And when we support ourselves with a diet plentiful in vegetables, especially by *replacing* sugary and starchy foods with those vegetables, we promote our internal bodily environment to be more alkaline. A more alkaline body, as opposed to a sugar-filled acidic one, supports the immune system and the nervous system among others, as well as reduces and virtually, eliminates any potential breeding grounds for bacteria, pathogens, and cancers. They just cannot survive in it.

So it is true what they say, you are what you eat! As pertaining to insulin resistance, let it be known that vegetables are one food group that is virtually completely safe. Just watch out for starchy vegetables like potatoes as well as sweeter vegetables like beets and carrots and consider their relevance to the severity of the insulin resistant condition. Again, monitor blood testing a few hours after eating these specific foods.

Fats

In the way of the healthy body, we all ideally require at minimum roughly 7% to 10% body fat. This recommendation comes from fat's ability to insulate the body to some degree, but more specifically it acts as a cushioned lining for internal organs in the abdomen. Fats also serve as energy stores within the body as a resource of necessity during endurance activities or simply when our regular blood sugar reserves have been depleted.

Perhaps you have heard that to start burning fat in a cardio workout, you must engage in some vigorous activity for at least 20 minutes leading up to it. That's to give you an idea that all it takes to burn up blood glucose reserves and start dipping into fat storage for energy is 20 minutes of constant movement.

Also known as lipids when speaking of fat cells in the body, we now know a few correlations between lipids and diabetes from the previous chapters that are worth reviewing here. One significant note is that 90% of people with type 2 diabetes were obese when diagnosed, so keeping fatty foods in the diet when making an earnest effort to recover is probably not a good idea.

Another red flag that should signal the avoidance of consuming fats in a state of insulin resistance is the buildup of lipids in the blood along with glucose because a lack of insulin prevents the removal of fat from the blood into storage lipid cells. Recall that plaque accumulation in blood vessels throughout the body constrains flow and can lead to serious complications from poor or nonexistent circulation in certain areas, preventing the ability to heal from even minor scrapes.

There are certain kinds of fats to discern from that can be good for you and those that are bad for you. Regardless of which side of the fence they come from, any type of fat should still be consumed in moderation, so whether you may be insulin resistant or not, keep in mind the daily recommended values, consultation from a medical professional that you trust, and the serving size of that particular food.

It is important to consult with a medical professional about consuming fats with regards to an insulin resistant condition because what may be recommended depends on the severity of the disorder and there are certain fats that support bodily function. Oftentimes talk about fats lump them all together in a "bad" category and should be avoided or eaten sparingly, but that is perhaps only because the types of fatty foods that are most popular and readily available are bad. This is in reference to trans and saturated fats, which cause higher levels of LDLs (low-density lipoproteins) that manifest as cholesterol and plaque, sticking to arterial and coronary walls. Trans fats result from the conversion of liquid oil to a solid, known as hydrogenation. These types of fats are recognized as being solid at room temperature and are usually found in meats, dairy products, and hydrogenated oils.

On the other hand, eating poly and monounsaturated fats as well as foods rich in Omega-3 fats cause higher levels of HDLs (high-density lipoproteins) that help to remove sticky plaque from blood vessel walls, lubricate joints and muscles, as well as nourish the skin. Unsaturated fats are typically liquid at room temperature with an oily texture. They can be found in many plant products and cold pressed oils. Below you can see the distinction of more examples between good and bad fats.

Trans and Saturated fats: beef and other cow meats; pork and other pig meats; lamb; whole milk; butter; most cheeses; margarine; deep-fried foods; partially hydrogenated oils found in commercially baked pastries, doughnuts, and cookies; candy; crackers and other packaged snack foods; many processed foods

Poly and Mono Unsaturated fats: fish such as tuna, mackerel, trout, sockeye salmon, flounder, herring and sardines; first cold pressed oils (look for it on the label) like olive, sesame, flax and safflower; nuts and nut butters like peanuts, almonds, macadamias, walnuts and pecans; seeds like flax, sesame and pumpkin; avocado

Is there any inferencing going on here? It becomes evident that most manufactured products should be avoided altogether or at the very least reduced in consumption while natural foods and less commercially farmed fish are better for the body. This should better reflect the condition of the options that food stores provide us with. Let's be honest with our bodies and provide them with the natural nourishment that Earth intended for us, because commercial and chemically manufactured food is literally making us sick.

It is a really good idea and would be to your benefit as well as everyone else's to make a habit of reading nutritional labels on food products.

Proteins

Protein is *the* central nutrient that is essential to every cell in the body. It comprises hair, it is used by the body to build or generate and repair tissues, and also aids in the production of enzymes such as those in the saliva and stomach to digest foods as well as hormones that help to regulate bodily functions (*such as insulin production*). Protein also serves a role as the fodder for creating bone tissues, muscle fibers, cartilage, skin, and blood.

Combined with fats and carbohydrates they form a macronutrient, meaning that the body requires fairly large amounts of it. Unlike fats and carbohydrates, however, there are no reserves of protein to pull from when the body needs more of it. So it becomes our responsibility to incorporate a steady amount of protein in our diets without exceeding portions, which happens to average out to about 4 ounces of meat per meal as one example. According to doctors, this figure can vary depending on age, sex, and level of activity in one's life.

In the case of insulin resistance and depending on the severity of an individual case, we have seen that unchecked diabetes can result in the body converting protein in the body to glucose for energy as a last resort since it cannot uptake it from blood reserves and has already burned up the body's fat stores.

This means the energy is coming from broken down protein in muscles, causing them to weaken and atrophy as well as other areas of the body like hair, leading to hair loss. Protein breakdown into glucose actually takes twice as long for the body to process and requires more effort, putting additional strain on organ systems.

So when it comes to rebuilding a weakened body after the disorder has been diagnosed and you or someone you know starts on the path to recovery, there should be no doubt that protein sources should play a central role in the diet. Similar to getting wise about fat consumption, where you get your protein from can greatly determine the progress or backstepping of the healing process.

No hot dog and bacon tango here. Eating large quantities of these processed meats along with deli meats has actually been linked to the increased risk of type 2 diabetes and cardiovascular disease. Just coming from that road, we know there is no need to take a different path to the same alarming place.

Below is a list of great food sources to get protein from, and vegan/vegetarian readers will be pleased to discover if you were not already aware that meats do not even make up the majority of the list.

Protein sources:

Fish, the same as those listed in the healthy fat category.

> Poultry, which contains most of the saturated fat in the skin that can be removed.

> Beans, combined with corn or grains like rice, become a complete protein. They are also chock-full of fiber that will stave off hunger pains and help you feel full until your next meal.

> Nuts, a high source of protein that is near-comparable to red meats, so watch your portions!

> Whole grains, especially sprouted whole grains, providing you with protein plus fiber.

Now just to dispel a common misconception, the term "build muscle" is not 100% accurate to describe what is actually happening. We never actually generate more muscle fibers to become stronger or beef up when it comes to weight lifting. What is actually happening is the micro-scarring of pre-existing muscle fibers when exercising and lifting weights.

This explains the relative soreness felt the day after a workout. Protein's role here comes in *repairing* those broken down muscle tissues, and as those tissues are repeatedly broken down and then repaired with micro scars they increase in volume, resulting in larger, stronger muscles. This may be handy to know when rebuilding weakened muscles.

Speaking of workouts, the following is a little formula to abide by to provide optimal conditions for the body so you can get a quality workout and properly restore necessary nutrients. Since you are going to be expending an above average amount of energy, it is helpful to eat a meal at least thirty minutes ahead or a snack right beforehand that consists of a greater portion of carbs (the complex kind) for extra energy with a smaller portion of protein for sustainability. Immediately after your workout it is beneficial to resupply the body with a greater portion of protein to help the body repair itself with a smaller portion of carbs to replenish all the energy you have just expended.

Chapter 5: Extra Tips to Getting Your Health and Energy Back

This chapter is dedicated to tips, tricks, strategies to end tragedies like reverting back to pitfall habits, as well as a few other golden sage words of advice. After reading this chapter it is my hope that you will feel confident and well-equipped to take your life back and live it even better than before.

We can start off by resetting your perception to one of empowerment, growth, and gratitude: consider that you or someone you know who may be showing signs or has already been diagnosed with insulin resistance has only reached this point to gain a deeper understanding of oneself.

You have been given the opportunity, as serious as it may seem, to take a closer look at certain life habits that are no longer working for you. Whether they may be rooted in the physical realm pertaining to diet and inactivity, the emotional realm concerning accumulated stress or trauma, or the psychological realm as a matter of a confining or resistant perspective toward life, this crossroads is offering you an opening to become aware of some deeper aspect to change for the better. And that 'better' can be a no-holds-barred chance to shape your life exactly the way you see fit, exploring and manifesting the innermost *feel-good* desires that perhaps you have put on the backburner for long enough now.

So I encourage you to take this chance, step through this open door, and let's get you back to a true sense of yourself in your own personal power. This ain't gonna be no gym jockey, pusher-man course of intensity riding you along – we're going to progress at your own gentle pace, recognizing the value of the process every baby step of the way.

Exercise

Here is a tip off to the game: see it as something fun – you are doing it for yourself, and you are totally worth the effort. Another mindful note is to monitor your glucose levels closely: check them before every meal and workout, remembering the foods that raise blood glucose and that exercise lowers it.

Now for the following information, let's emphasize a few key points regarding the body's natural and integrated systems. The first is that blood circulation should be a primary focal point. It brings oxygen and nutrients to every cell in the body and removes metabolic wastes and carbon dioxide that contribute to acidic pH levels from every cell so that they can maintain peak performance of health.

That's why in association with every workout, and really every day, stretching is very important. A good stretch means that you are moving slowly into it breathing deeply and evenly until you reach your threshold and then extend just past your comfort zone, continuing the same breath pattern for at least a few breaths, and then maintaining that pattern as you move slowly out of that position.

Stretch lightly to engage the muscles before a workout and more deeply after a workout to promote better circulation and open up the muscles and joints more.

The next point is your pace. Do not rush; it is a misplaced epidemic of our society. Take your time to start out slowly and get the movement of the exercise right the first time and with each repetition afterwards. This way you will become more aware of the natural movement of your body at the joints and you will develop better body mechanics and posture, which relieves stress on the joints and internal organs. You will also avoid straining and banging your muscles and joints, giving you a better quality workout. Start slowly, find the controlled pace that works for you, and with time and consistency you will develop speed with precision.

A following key point has already been discussed in chapter 3 about synchronizing breath with the movement. It promotes body awareness, improved blood circulation, physical and mental ease, as well as cleaner, healthier cells. Breathe from the diaphragm, the muscle that actually expands the lungs, located just below the ribcage. Your inhale should see the upper abdomen expand outward while your exhale should see it fall back into place again.

Some practices have you inhale into every movement and exhale out of it while others have you do it the other way around. As long as your breath is synchronized with the movement that is all that really matters. Now let's get into it.

Strength training: The form of exercise here will depend on how much you have already been affected by the insulin resistance disorder. We will cover basic principles of body movement and mechanics that you can then alter for yourself with weights.

Consider that almost every muscle in the body attaches at two points over a joint. In common physical therapy practices, their exercises have you isolate one group of muscles at a time by enforcing this particular principal. In weight training and strength building it is called "isometrics". You can search these topics online for specific movements.

Cardio: These exercises coordinate rapid and consistent movement with the lungs and the heart rate. They get your blood pumping to give you a good body cleanout of wastes through circulation and perspiration. They strengthen and regulate your heart, as well as build endurance in the muscles and lungs (diaphragm), toning and strengthening them too.

Strong lung power means deeper breaths, reducing shallow breathing, which means healthier blood and cells which means more energy for you throughout your day to work with.

Common cardio exercises are running, jogging, rowing machine, swimming, jump rope, stair-stepping and bicycling to name a few.

Remember that cardio exercise only need be 20 to 30 minutes per day or every other day *for a healthy person*. With diabetes, you should start out very gradually at one to two times per week until you know exactly how it affects you.

Yoga: Contrary to popular belief, yoga began long ago as a philosophy and way of life rather than a series of stretches and poses. Only within the past 70 or so years with increased popularity has yoga become what it is commonly known for today. There are many forms and styles of yoga that are well worth researching because there seems to be a type suited for all different kinds of people. The most common form seen in mainstream is called Vinyasa Yoga.

These poses and stretches come with several benefits. Some are as simple as providing effective stretches for every part of the body that range from light to very deep, as well as shaping and toning the muscles. Other benefits include better circulation, a healthier and sharper nervous system, stress reduction (both physical and mental), all the way to tapping into a sense of something greater than ourselves that fuels our desires and inspires us for the greater good.

Yoga poses to do at home and local yoga centers if you so wish to join a class can also be easily found online. For home tryouts I recommend starting with "Sun Salutation" sets: there are different adaptations for different experience levels so find one that suits you. They are gentle, succinct, and complete.

Others: I highly recommend at least looking into some form of Tai Chi or Qi Gong. These practices are typically confused as exercises for elderly people, although that is simply because elders usually deal with weakened muscles, joint pain, a relatively inactive lifestyle and poor circulation (sound familiar?). The truth is every single person can benefit from these practices and the younger one starts, the deeper one can go into the underlying principles of these smooth, gentle and relaxing movements.

How to Deal with Cravings

The short and straight piece of advice here is DO NOT KEEP CRAVED FOODS AND BEVERAGES IN THE HOME. Out of sight, out of mind really does work. Obviously, when living with other people who have different, less restrictive diets that choose to keep such craved foods around, this can be more difficult. You can try having these products stored in a place where you will not see them.

You can also try to associate these products with an object of disgust that is personal to you and attach a picture of that object on the product. For example, if you despise cigarettes but you have become attached to soda and there are bottles in the fridge or pantry, you can tape a picture of a blackened, ashy cigarette or a whole overflowing ashtray of them onto the soda bottles. The truth is that they are both equally damaging to the body.

Educating yourself repetitively and reminding yourself of all the adverse effects that are caused by said craved food or beverage is always an option. Anytime you feel a craving you can remind yourself because of these complications that it is not really worth it and you do not really want it.

Moving your perspective ahead to where you really want to transition from this stage in life, when you feel a craving coming on you can take a deep breath, sit with it for a minute without acting upon it and confirm to yourself that yes, indulging would be a temporary solution. Then take another deep breath in this moment of stillness and focus, asking yourself, "What do I *really* want out of the future, and what does my life look like without this thing?"

Cravings, like addictions, are part chemical dependency within the body and they are part mental by associative attachment in some way. The trick is to identify the attachment by understanding the nature of your association with it and within that realization, which often feels like an epiphany of sorts, breaking the attachment and ushering forth a truer, stronger, healthier desire that benefits you both now and later on.

This last method starts stepping into the realm of mind control and hypnosis techniques that have proven over decades to be very effective for people who were open to just trying it and truly wanting to quit. There are several videos and professionals to be found online who practice and help others, so you might consider it worth checking out.

Sleep

Sleep is a natural part of life because it provides us with the rest and rejuvenation that the body and mind need to be prepared for all that life has to bring the following day. It is so important that entire books have been written on the subject, dedicated to exploring its implications and relevance so please do not equate the brevity of this section to the worth of this activity. It is indeed an activity of a different kind even though it may seem like we are doing nothing.

There are five stages of sleep, each relating to a different state of consciousness, the fourth of which pertains to the deepest form of sleep when we are fully unconscious. Stage IV sleep as it is medically known is when the body takes the time to repair itself on a cellular level. For a person trying to heal from an illness, the importance of spending the required amount of time in this stage is magnified multifold.

Unfortunately, due the state of society we live in these days, stage IV sleep is also the most deprived. It can be attributed to late night entertainment in the forms of TV, movies, social media, internet perusing, and smartphones just to name a few. Lights in the bedroom, even tiny ones from electronic devices, affect our quality of sleep and prevent us from reaching stage IV.

Some useful advice here is to firmly establish the bedroom as what it was meant for. Do not bring any electronics into the bedroom, especially after dark except for an alarm for the morning. Do not bring any work into the bedroom. It is a psychological tactic that has proven to be quite effective for those people with sleep troubles. Make the bedroom's sole purpose for rest and valuable sleep time.

Water

As another crucial element to our daily existence, water is what lubricates all the systems of the body and keeps us functioning properly. Being dehydrated causes us to become irritable, cloud-minded, confused, tense and sub-operational. We keep hearing experts say that we are composed of 90% water or more, so it only goes to show that we should stay that way by making sure that we keep hydrated.

The proper amount of water to consume daily is eight cups. Due to polyuria and compensated circulation, people with insulin resistance should consume a bit more, about 10 to 12 cups of water every day. When we talk about water consumption, we are talking strictly about a glass filled with nothing else. We are not referring to tea, coffee, Kool-Aid or sports drinks; they do not get absorbed in the body in the same way. Speaking of absorption, it is ideal for digestion to prime this system's organs for ease of proper food intake and nutrient absorption by drinking a glass of water a half-hour in advance of eating.

There are so many factors that dehydrate us to be aware of that not all of them can be listed here, however, the following will provide you with some examples of dehydration-inducing products to avoid. We should all avoid these or at the very least reduce our consumption of them to sparing amounts, yet it goes doubly so for those with insulin resistance.

Dehydrators: Sugar and sugary foods, cigarettes, coffee (also a diuretic, causing us to have to urinate more and thus lose body water), sports drinks containing electrolytes (sources of excessive amounts of potassium, sodium and other nutrients that effectually tax the body's organs over time).

Stress

Stress is such a gravely under-emphasized factor in mainstream medical practice that often serves as the root of most disorders because again the common Western medical approach to illness is to address the symptoms rather than the underlying causes. It has yet to see the human dynamic as a holistic composite of physicality in intimate connection with the ever-present yet seldom attributed emotional aspect, as well as the psychological component of the particular nature of an individual's thoughts and perspective.

Together, these components shape our individual reality, which all add into determining our overall health through varying levels of consciousness. That is why it is so beneficial to take it upon ourselves in becoming as aware as we are capable of being, noticing our personal patterns of cause and effect, stimulus and response, as well as thoughts and reactions.

There is a phenomenon known as *somatic emotional release* that is sometimes seen in massage therapy and has proven this intimate connection between the body, emotions and thoughts. We all have the potential of experiencing it at varying degrees, although it is often seen more prominently in people who have experienced some kind of emotional trauma. "Soma" is the Latin name for "body", and this particular phenomenon refers to the understanding that unresolved emotions can be stored in the cellular memory of the body.

Extracting this understanding shown by the somatic emotional concept gives way to the evidence that physical diseases manifesting within the body and presenting any number of symptoms are deeply linked to suppressed emotions that resulted from some original stressful situation. The body remembers it and requires resolution still, even if the mind had forgotten or the person refused to properly acknowledge it.

That's why I mentioned at the top of this chapter that being faced with a physically manifested illness of the body can be viewed as a blessing in disguise, providing us with an opportunity to look deeper within so that we may go forward and grow exponentially. We have the power within us, educating ourselves gives us the tools, and together it is time now to let it out. Find your personal healthy outlet to release the stress and embrace fulfillment in its wake.

Supplements

We can take a straight shot here at listing the beneficial supplements that help insulin resistance. Since diabetes can be related and lead to other complications such as candidiasis, some of these supplements will cover ground for them too.

Fish oils – contain Omega-3 fatty acids

Turmeric – reduces inflammation

Ginger – reduces inflammation and soothes digestive organs

Wild Reishi Extract – supports and enhances immune system function

Pancreatin – aids in the digestion of proteins, carbs, and fats

Digestive enzymes – supports the digestion and absorption of proteins, carbs, fiber and fats

Boswellia – a.k.a. the Indian version of frankincense used for thousands of years for inflammation reduction as well as treating arthritis, diarrhea, and pulmonary disease

Gynostemma tea and Spring Dragon Extract – both powerful adaptogens that smooth out the stress response system to provide relief for the adrenal glands and promote an increase in healthy immune system functions

Conclusion

I hope this book was able to help you to find your way through the potentially fearful terrain of waking up to, temporarily living with, and moving past a state of insulin resistance. With the steps outlined in this book as a guide, you won't become another statistic. You will join the pioneering ranks of leading others into a deeper understanding of just what illness is and how previously conceived lifelong illnesses can be reversed.

The next step is to be patient with the process and stay true to the regimen you have created for yourself according to these guidelines. During this time, make it a daily practice to envision what your life looks like after the healing process is completed. Trust it, reinforce it, and believe it whole-heartedly to be true. Your thoughts determine your reality.

Thank you and good luck!

www.ingramcontent.com/pod-product-compliance
Lightning Source LLC
Chambersburg PA
CBHW070408190526
45169CB00003B/1161